Veg Mediterranean Diet

The Meal Prep Cookbook, Easy and Healthy Meals to Cook, Prepare, Grab and Go

Healthy Kitchen

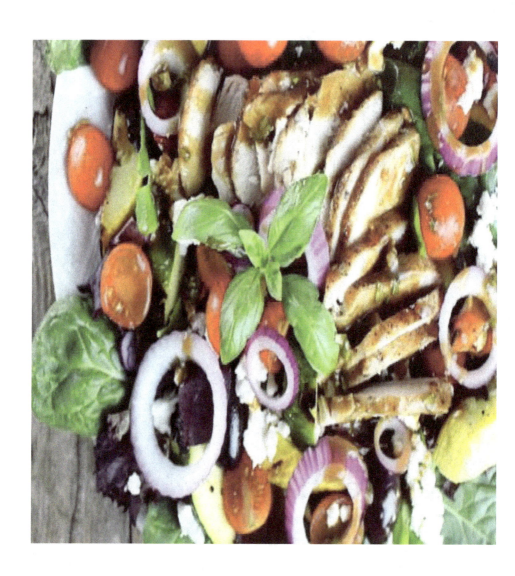

© Copyright 2020 by Healthy Kitchen- All rights reserved.

The following Book is reproduced below with the goal of providing information that is as accurate and reliable as possible. Regardless, purchasing this Book can be seen as consent to the fact that both the publisher and the author of this book are in no way experts on the topics discussed within and that any recommendations or suggestions that are made herein are for entertainment purposes only. Professionals should be consulted as needed prior to undertaking any of the action endorsed herein.

This declaration is deemed fair and valid by both the American Bar Association and the Committee of Publishers Association and is legally binding throughout the United States.

Furthermore, the transmission, duplication, or reproduction of any of the following work including specific information will be considered an illegal act irrespective of if it is done electronically or in print. This extends to creating a secondary or tertiary copy of the work or a recorded copy and is only allowed with the express written consent from the Publisher. All additional right reserved.

The information in the following pages is broadly considered a truthful and accurate account of facts and as such, any inattention, use, or misuse of the information in question by the reader will render any resulting actions solely under their purview. There are no scenarios in which the publisher or the original author of this work can be in any fashion deemed liable for any hardship or damages that may befall them after undertaking information described herein.

Additionally, the information in the following pages is intended only for informational purposes and should thus be thought of as universal. As befitting its nature, it is presented without assurance regarding its prolonged validity or interim quality. Trademarks that are mentioned are done without written consent and can in no way be considered an endorsement from the trademark holder.

Sommario

INTRODUCTION 9
- The Mediterranean Diet's History 9
- Start your Diet 9
- Losing Weight 15
- Spring Sandwich 16
- Springtime Quinoa Salad 18
- Honey and Vanilla Custard Cups with Crunchy Filo Pastry 20
- Mediterranean Tostadas 22
- Vegetable Ratatouille 24
- Citrus Cups 26
- Mixed Berry Pancakes and Ricotta 28
- Mediterranean Frittata 30
- Caponata 31
- Mediterranean Style Fruit Medley 34
- Mediterranean Watermelon Salad 35
- Melon Cucumber Smoothie 36
- Peanut Banana Yogurt Bowl 37
- Pomegranate and Lychee Sorbet 38
- Pomegranate Granita with Lychee 39
- Roasted Berry and Honey Yogurt Pops 40
- Scrumptious Cake with Cinnamon 41
- Smoothie Bowl with Dragon Fruit 42
- Soothing Red Smoothie 43
- Strawberry and Avocado Medley 44
- Strawberry Banana Greek Yogurt Parfaits 45
- Summertime Fruit Salad 46
- Sweet Tropical Medley Smoothie 47
- Spinach and Grilled Feta Salad 48

Creamy Cool Salad	49
Broccoli Salad with Caramelized Onions	50
Baked Cauliflower Mixed Salad	51
Quick Arugula Salad	52
Bell Pepper and Tomato Salad	53
One Bowl Spinach Salad	54
Olive and Red Bean Salad	55
Fresh and Light Cabbage Salad	56
Vegetable Patch Salad	57
Cucumber Greek yoghurt Salad	58
Chickpea Salad Recipe	59
Orange salad	60
Yogurt lettuce salad recipe	61
Fruit de salad recipe	62
Chickpea with mint salad recipe	63
Grapy Fennel salad	64
Greenie salad recipe	65
A Refreshing Detox Salad	66
Amazingly Fresh Carrot Salad	67
Anchovy and Orange Salad	68
Arugula with Blueberries 'n Almonds	70
Asian Peanut Sauce Over Noodle Salad	71
Vegetable Fritters	73
Asian Salad with pistachios	74
Balela Salad from the Middle East	76
Blue Cheese and Portobello Salad	78
Blue Cheese and Arugula Salad	80
Broccoli Salad Moroccan Style	81
Classic Greek Salad	82

Cold Zucchini Noodle Bowl	83
Coleslaw Asian Style	86
Cucumber and Tomato Salad	88
Cucumber Salad Japanese Style	89
Easy Garden Salad with Arugula	90
Easy Quinoa & Pear Salad	91
Easy-Peasy Club Salad	93
Fennel and Seared Scallops Salad	94
Fruity Asparagus-Quinoa Salad	96
Garden Salad with Balsamic Vinegar	98
Rice with Vermicelli	99
Fava Beans and Rice	100
Buttered Fava Beans	101
Freekeh	102
Fried Rice Balls with Tomato Sauce	103
Spanish-Style Rice	105
Zucchini with Rice and Tzatziki	107
Cannellini Beans with Rosemary and Garlic Aioli	109
Jeweled Rice	110
Asparagus Risotto	112
Vegetable Paella	114
Eggplant and Rice Casserole	116
Many Vegetable Couscous	118
Kushari	120
Bulgur with Tomatoes and Chickpeas	123
Cauliflower Steaks with Olive Citrus Sauce	125
Pistachio Mint Pesto Pasta	127

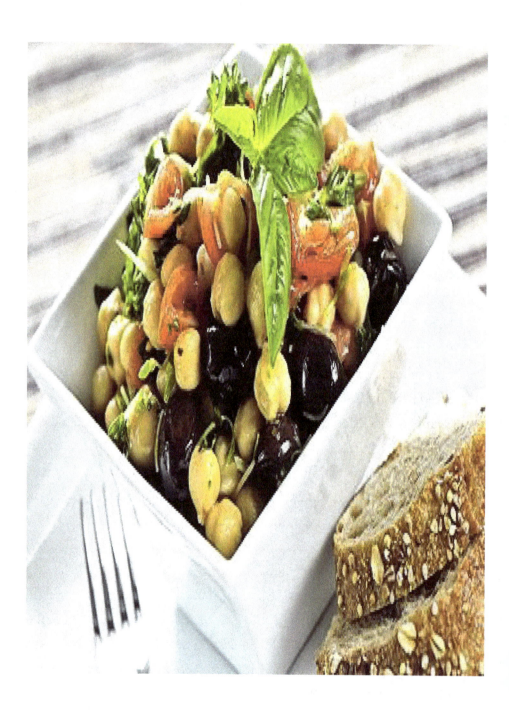

INTRODUCTION

The Mediterranean Diet's History

While this diet was first brought to light in 1945, until the 1990s, when people started to grow a newfound knowledge of what they were eating, it did not really reach mainstream levels. This is about the time when fitness programs started to surface on TV and healthy eating started to become popular again. The Mediterranean diet is based on the premise that there is a much lower risk of heart disease among people in these regions than in people with comparable fat consumption in other areas of the world. For instance, year after year, a person living in the United States and a person living in Greece might consume the exact same amount of fat, but the American would have a greater risk of suffering from heart disease because certain elements of his or her diet are missing.

Start your Diet

Stay Hydrated

Once you've started and are fully immersed in the Mediterranean diet, you might notice that you've started to feel a little bit weak, and a little bit colder, than you're used to. The Mediterranean diet places an emphasis on trying to cut out as much sodium from your diet as possible, which is very healthy for some of us who already have high sodium levels. Sodium, obviously is found in salt, and so we proceed to cut out salt – and then drink enough water to drain every last drop of sodium from our bodies. When it comes to hydration, the biological mechanisms for keeping us saturated and quenched rely on an equal balance of sodium and potassium. Sodium can be found in your interstitial fluid, and potassium can be found inside our cytoplasm – two sides of one wall. When you drink tons of water, sweat a lot at the gym, or both, your sodium leaves your body in your urine and your sweat. Potassium, on the other hand, is only really lost through the urine – and even then, it's rare. This means that our bodies almost constantly need a refill on our sodium levels.

Vitamins and Supplements

Vitamins and minerals can be found in plants and animals, yes, but more often than not fruits and vegetables are much stronger sources. When consume another animal, we are consuming the sum total of all of the energy and nutrition that that animal has also consumed. This might sound like a sweet deal, but the pig you're eating used that energy in his own daily life, and therefore only has a tiny bit left to offer you. Plants, on the other hand, are first-hand sources of things like calcium, vitamin K, and vitamin C, which our bodies require daily doses of.

Meal Preparation and Portion Planning

If you haven't heard of the term "meal prep" before now, it's a beautiful day to learn something that will save you time, stress, and inches on your waistline. Meal prep, short for meal preparation, is a habit that was developed mostly by the body building community in order to accurately track your macronutrients. The basic idea behind meal prep is that each weekend, you manage your free time around cooking and preparing all of your meals for the upcoming week. While most meal preppers do their grocery shopping and

cooking on Sundays, to keep their meals the freshest, you can choose to cook on a Saturday if that works better with your schedule. Meal prep each week uses one large grocery list of bulk ingredients to get all the supplies you need to make four dinners and four lunches of your choice. This means that you might have to do a bit of mental math quadrupling the serving size, but all you have to do is multiply each ingredient by four. Although you don't have to meal prep more than one meal with four portions each week, if you're already in the kitchen, you most likely have cooking time to work on something else.

Tracking Your Macronutrients

Wouldn't it be nice if you could have a full nutritional label for each of your home-cooked meals, just to make sure that your numbers are adding up in favor of weight loss? Oddly enough, tracking your macronutrients in order to calculate the nutritional value of each of your meals and portions is as easy as stepping on the scale. Not the scale in your bathroom, however. A food scale! If you've never had a good relationship with your weight and numbers, you might suddenly find that they aren't too bad after all. Food scales are used to measure, well, your food, but there's a slick system of online calculators and fitness applications for your smart phone that can take this number and turn it into magic. When you meal prep each week, keep track of your recipes diligently. Remember how you multiplied each of the ingredients on the list by four to create four servings? You're going to want to remember how much of each vegetable, fruit, grain, nut, and fat you cooked with. While you wait for your meal to finish cooking, find a large enough plastic container to fit all of your meals. Make sure it's clean and dry, and use the empty container to zero out your scale.

Counting Calories and Forming a Deficit

When it comes down to the technical science, there is one way and only one way to lose weight: by eating fewer calories in one day than your body requires to survive. Now, this doesn't mean that you can't lose weight for other reasons – be it water weight, as a result of stress, or simply working out harder. Although counting calories might not be the most fun way to lose weight, a calorie deficit is the only sure-fire way of guaranteeing that you reap all the weight loss benefits of the Mediterranean diet for your efforts. Scientifically, you already know that the healthy rate of weight loss for the average adult is between one and two pounds per week.

Get ready for a little bit more math, but it's nothing you can't handle in the name of a smaller waistline. One pound of fat equals around thirty-five hundred Calories, which means that your caloric deficit needs to account for that number, each week, without making too much of a dent on your regular nutrition. For most of us, we're used to eating between fifteen hundred and two thousand calories per day, which gives you a blessedly simply five hundred calorie deficit per day in order to reach your healthy weight loss goals. If you cut out exactly five hundred calories each day, you should be able to lose one pound of fat by the end of seven days. Granted, this estimate does take into account thirty minutes of daily exercise, but the results are still about the same when you rely on the scientific facts. If your age, height, weight, and sex predispose you to eat either more or less calories per day, you might want to consult with your doctor about the healthiest way for you to integrate a caloric deficit into your Mediterranean diet.

Goal Setting to Meet Your Achievements

On the subject of control, there are a few steps and activities that you should go through before you begin your Mediterranean diet just to make sure that you have clear and realistic goals in mind. Sitting down to set goals before embarking on a totally new diet routine will help you stay focused and committed during your Mediterranean diet. While a Mediterranean diet lifestyle certainly isn't as demanding as some of the crazy diet fads you see today, it can be a struggle to focus on eating natural fruits and vegetables that are more "salt of the Earth" foods than we're used to. You already know that when it comes to weight loss, you shouldn't expect to lose more than one to two pounds per week healthily while you're dieting. You are still welcome to set a weight loss goal with time in mind, but when it comes to the Mediterranean diet, you should set your goals for one month in the future.

Losing Weight

Further studies have provided examples of weight loss from the Mediterranean diet, as 322 individuals participated in an experiment where some individuals were exposed to a low-carb diet, others undertook a low-fat diet, and some consumed only a Mediterranean diet. The findings found that those on the Mediterranean diet had the greatest weight loss of all with 12 and 10 pounds respectively being lost by the top two participants. The study stressed that weight loss from the Mediterranean diet is successful and should be considered by anyone who has difficulty losing weight.

Spring Sandwich

Ingredients:

- 1 pinch of salt
- 1 pinch of black pepper
- 4 teaspoons of extra-virgin olive oil
- 4 eggs
- 4 multigrain sandwich thins
- 1 onion, finely diced
- 1 tomato, sliced thinly
- 2 cups of fresh baby spinach leaves
- 4 tablespoons of crumbled feta
- 1 sprig of fresh rosemary

Directions:

1. Preheat your oven to 375 F .
2. Slice the multigrain sandwich thins open and brush each side with one teaspoon of olive oil. Place them into the oven and toast for five minutes. Remove and set aside.
3. Situate non-stick skillet over medium heat, add the remaining 2 teaspoons of olive oil and strip the leaves of rosemary off into the pan. Add in the eggs, one by one.
4. Cook until the eggs have whitened, and the yolks stay runny. Flip once using a spatula and then remove from the heat.

5. Place the multigrain thins onto serving plates, then place the spinach leaves on top, followed by sliced tomato, one egg, and a sprinkling of feta cheese. Add salt and pepper, then close your sandwich using the remaining multigrain thins.

Springtime Quinoa Salad

Ingredients:

<u>for vinaigrette:</u>

- 1 pinch of salt
- 1 pinch of black pepper
- ½ teaspoon of dried thyme
- ½ teaspoon of dried oregano
- ¼ cup of extra-virgin olive oil
- 1 tablespoon of honey
- juice of 1 lemon
- 1 clove of garlic, minced
- 2 tablespoons of fresh basil, diced

<u>for salad:</u>

- 1 ½ cups of cooked quinoa
- 4 cups of mixed leafy greens
- ½ cup of kalamata olives, halved and pitted
- ¼ cup of sun-dried tomatoes, diced
- ½ cup of almonds, raw, unsalted and diced

Directions:

1. Combine all the vinaigrette ingredients together, either by hand or using a blender or food processor. Set the vinaigrette aside in the refrigerator.
2. In a large salad bowl, combine the salad ingredients.
3. Drizzle the vinaigrette over the salad, then serve.

Honey and Vanilla Custard Cups with Crunchy Filo Pastry

Ingredients:

- 1 vanilla bean, cut lengthways
- 2 cups of full-fat milk
- 1/3 cup of honey
- 1 tablespoon of brown sugar
- 2 tablespoons of custard powder
- 4 to 6 ripe figs, quartered
- 1 sheet of filo pastry
- 2 tablespoons of raw pistachios

Directions:

1. Situate saucepan over medium heat, simmer vanilla bean, milk, and honey
2. In a heatproof dish, combine the sugar and custard powder. Transfer the milk mixture into the bowl containing the custard powder. Using a whisk, combine well and then transfer back into the saucepan.
3. Bring to a boil, constantly whisking until the custard thickens. Remove the vanilla bean.
4. Pour the custard into cups and allow to chill in the refrigerator for 2 hours.

5. Heat your oven to 350 F and line a baking tray with parchment.
6. Put the pastry sheet onto an even surface and spray lightly with olive oil cooking spray.
7. Sprinkle half the pistachios over the pastry and then fold the pastry in half. Heat up 2 tablespoons of honey in the microwave, then coat the pastry.
8. Place the pastry into the oven and allow to bake for 10 minutes. Remove from heat and allow it to cool.
9. Gently break the filo pastry into pieces, then top the custard with the shards and fresh-cut figs.

Mediterranean Tostadas

Ingredients:

- 1 pinch salt
- 1 pinch black pepper
- 1 pinch oregano
- 1 pinch garlic powder
- 4 tostadas
- 1 tablespoon of extra-virgin olive oil
- ½ cup of milk
- ½ cup of roasted red pepper hummus
- 8 eggs, beaten
- ½ cup of green onion, finely diced
- ½ cup of red bell peppers, finely diced
- ½ cup of diced cucumber
- ½ cup of diced tomato
- ¼ cup of crumbled feta
- 1 handful of fresh basil

Directions:

1. Position non-stick skillet over medium heat, cook olive oil and red peppers. Cook until these have softened, then

add the salt, pepper, oregano, garlic powder, milk, eggs, and onion.
2. Gently stir the mixture until you reach a scrambled egg consistency.
3. Once cooked through, remove from the heat.
4. Place a tostada onto each place, and top with the hummus, egg, tomato, cucumber, feta, and fresh basil leaves.

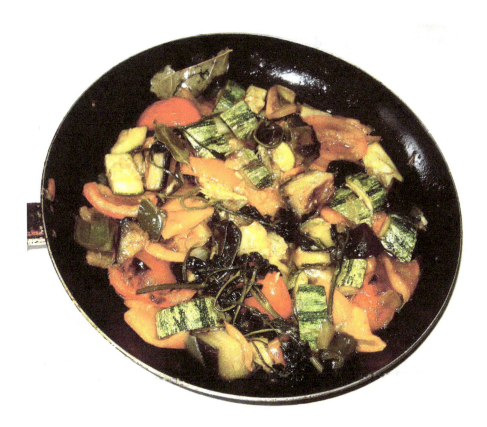

Vegetable Ratatouille

Ingredients:

- 1 pinch salt
- 1 pinch black pepper
- 1 pinch brown sugar
- ¼ cup extra-virgin olive oil
- ¼ cup of white wine
- 3 cloves of garlic
- 1 onion, diced
- 1 lb. of eggplant
- 1 cup of zucchini
- 1 ½ cups of canned tomato
- 1 red bell pepper, diced
- 1 green bell pepper, diced
- ½ cup of fresh basil

Directions:

1. Place saucepan over medium heat, cook olive oil and finely diced garlic and onion.
2. Add the cubed eggplant and continue to cook for a further 5 minutes.

3. Add the salt, pepper, and diced bell peppers. Allow to cook for another 3 minutes.
4. Add the sliced zucchini to the saucepan and cook for 3 minutes.
5. Mix white wine and canned tomatoes.
6. Allow to simmer for another five minutes. Taste the ratatouille.
7. Pull away from the heat, add the basil, and serve with a side portion of barley or brown rice.

Citrus Cups

Ingredients:

- ½ cup of water
- 1 tablespoon of orange juice
- 3 cups of full-fat Greek yogurt
- 1 vanilla bean
- 1 ruby grapefruit
- 2 mandarins
- 1 orange
- 6 strips of mandarin rind
- 1/3 cup of powdered sugar
- 1 small handful of fresh mint leaves

Directions:

1. Slice open the vanilla bean lengthways and transfer the seeds into a medium saucepan. Add the pod to the saucepan as well, followed by the water, sugar, and mandarin rind.
2. Bring the mixture to a boil, then turn down to a simmer and cook for five minutes or until the syrup has thickened.

3. Allow to cool, remove the pod, and stir in the orange juice.
4. Pour the syrup over the sliced citrus fruits and allow to rest.
5. Dish the yogurt up into four bowls, top with the citrus and syrup, sprinkle with a bit of mint, then serve.

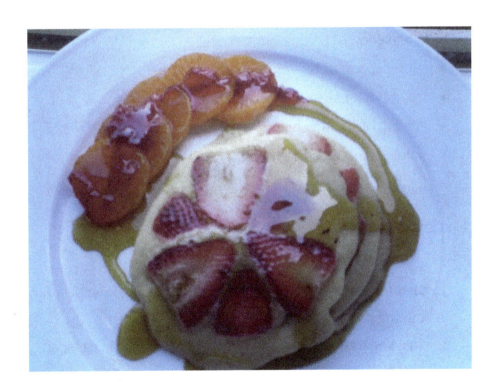

Mixed Berry Pancakes and Ricotta

Ingredients:

- 1 pinch of salt
- ½ cup of milk
- 1 tablespoon of canola oil
- 2 eggs
- 1 ½ tablespoon of coarse brown sugar
- 1 teaspoon of baking powder
- ¼ teaspoon of baking soda
- 1 1/3 cup of all-purpose flour
- ½ cup of ricotta cheese
- 1 cup of mixed berries

Directions:

1. In a mixing bowl, combine the salt, sugar, baking powder, baking soda, and flour.
2. In a separate mixing bowl, combine the ricotta, eggs, oil, and milk.
3. Combine the wet mixture with the dry mixture. Mix well. Put aside for 10 minutes.

4. Place a large, non-stick frying pan over medium heat. When the pan is hot to the touch, spoon even amounts of the batter into the pan, making sure that the batter dollops do not touch.
5. When they begin to bubble through, flip them over and cook for a further minute or two.
6. Follow this process until all the batter has been made into pancakes.
7. Evenly divide the pancakes between four plates. Top with mixed berries and drizzle with maple syrup and a few extra dollops of ricotta.

Mediterranean Frittata

Ingredients:

- 1 pinch of salt
- 1 pinch of black pepper
- 1 tablespoon of extra-virgin olive oil
- 2 egg whites
- 6 eggs
- 1 cup of goat cheese
- 1 cup of Parmesan, shredded
- 8 oz. of mixed mushrooms
- 1 leek, diced
- 1 lb. of asparagus, finely sliced
- ½ cup of fresh basil leaves

Directions:

1. Preheat your oven to 400 F.
2. Scourge egg whites and eggs, salt, pepper, Parmesan cheese, and basil leaves. Set this aside.

3. In a large skillet, preferably non-stick, add the olive oil and leeks over medium heat. Cook until the leeks have softened, then add in the mushrooms, asparagus, stir to combine and cook for a further 5 minutes.
4. Put egg mixture to the skillet, using a spatula to spread the eggs evenly over the mixture. Allow to cook for two minutes and then top with the goat cheese.
5. Place the skillet into the oven and allow to bake for five minutes
6. Remove from the oven and serve.

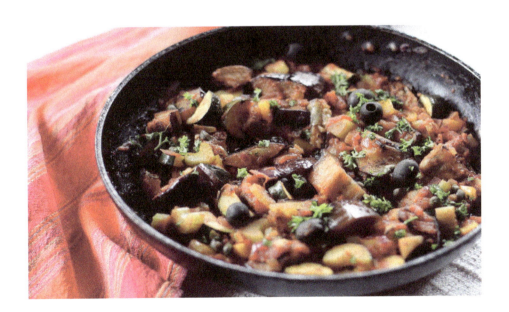

Caponata

Ingredients:

<u>for Caponata:</u>

- 1 pinch of salt
- 1 pinch of black pepper
- Fl oz. of extra-virgin olive oil
- Fl oz. of red wine vinegar
- 2 shallots, diced
- 4 sticks of celery, diced
- 4 plum tomatoes, diced
- 3 eggplants
- 2 teaspoons of capers
- oz. of raisins
- ½ cup of pine nuts, raw
- ½ cup of fresh basil leaves

<u>for bruschetta:</u>

- Extra-virgin olive oil
- 1 clove of garlic
- 8 slices of ciabatta

Directions:

1. Place casserole over medium heat, cook olive oil and cubed eggplant
2. Remove the eggplant and set aside.
3. Add the diced shallots to the casserole and cook until softened. Follow by adding the plum tomatoes.
4. Allow the tomatoes to break down and return the eggplant cubes to this mixture.
5. Add the salt, pepper, vinegar, celery, capers, and raisins.
6. Set heat to low, cover and simmer for 40 minutes. Once the vegetables have cooked through, remove from the heat and set aside.
7. Coat the sliced ciabatta with olive oil and place onto a griddle pan over medium heat. Remove once charred on both sides. Rub the ciabatta slices with garlic cloves to enhance their flavor.
8. Top the caponata with the pine nuts and basil leaves, and serve with the sliced ciabatta on the side.

Mediterranean Style Fruit Medley

Ingredients:

- 4 fuyu persimmons, sliced into wedges
- 1 ½ cups grapes, halved
- 8 mint leaves, chopped
- 1 tablespoon lemon juice
- 1 tablespoon honey
- ½ cups almond, toasted and chopped

Directions:

1. Combine all Ingredients in a bowl.
2. Toss then chill before serving.

Mediterranean Watermelon Salad

Ingredients:

- 6 cups mixed salad greens, torn
- 3 cups watermelon, seeded and cubed
- ½ cup onion, sliced
- 1 tablespoon extra-virgin olive oil
- 1/3 cup feta cheese, crumbled
- Cracked black pepper

Directions:

1. In a large bowl, mix all ingredients.
2. Toss to combine everything.
3. Allow to chill before serving.

Melon Cucumber Smoothie

Ingredients:

- ½ cucumber
- 2 slices of melon
- 2 tablespoons lemon juice
- 1 pear, peeled and sliced
- 3 fresh mint leaves
- ½ cup almond milk

Directions:

1. Place all Ingredients in a blender.
2. Blend until smooth.
3. Pour in a glass container and allow to chill in the fridge for at least 30 minutes.

Peanut Banana Yogurt Bowl

Ingredients:

- 4 cups Greek yogurt
- 2 medium bananas, sliced
- ¼ cup creamy natural peanut butter
- ¼ cup flax seed meal
- 1 teaspoon nutmeg

Directions:

1. Divide the yogurt between four bowls and top with banana, peanut butter, and flax seed meal.
2. Garnish with nutmeg.
3. Chill before serving.

Pomegranate and Lychee Sorbet

Ingredients:

- ¾ cup dragon fruit cubes
- 8 lychees, peeled and pitted
- Juice from 1 lemon
- 3 tablespoons stevia sugar
- 2 tablespoons pomegranate seeds

Directions:

1. In a blender, combine, the dragon fruit, lychees, lemon, and stevia sugar.
2. Pulse until smooth.
3. Pour the mixture in a container with lid and place inside the fridge.
4. Allow sorbet to harden for at least 8 hours.
5. Sprinkle with pomegranate seeds before serving.

Pomegranate Granita with Lychee

Ingredients:

- 500 millimeters pomegranate juice, organic and sugar-free
- 1 cup water
- ½ cup lychee syrup
- 2 tablespoons lemon juice
- 4 mint leaves
- 1 cup fresh lychees, pitted and sliced

Directions:

1. Place all Ingredients in a large pitcher.
2. Place inside the fridge to cool before serving.

Roasted Berry and Honey Yogurt Pops

Ingredients:

- 12 ounces mixed berries
- A dash of sea salt
- 2 tablespoons honey
- 2 cups whole Greek yogurt
- ½ small lemon, juice

Directions:

1. Preheat the oven to 3500F.
2. Line a baking sheet with parchment paper then set aside.
3. In a medium bowl, toss the berries with sea salt and honey.
4. Pour the berries on the prepared baking sheet.
5. Roast for 30 minutes while stirring halfway.
6. While the fruit is roasting, blend the Greek yogurt and lemon juice. Add honey to taste if desired.
7. Once the berries are done, cool for at least ten minutes.
8. Fold the berries into the yogurt mixture.
9. Pour into popsicle molds and allow to freeze for at least 8 hours.
10. Serve chilled.

Scrumptious Cake with Cinnamon

Ingredients:

- 1 lemon
- 4 eggs
- 1 tsp cinnamon
- ¼ lb. sugar
- ½ lb. ground almonds

Directions:

1. Preheat oven to 350oF. Then grease a cake pan and set aside.
2. On high speed, beat for three minutes the sugar and eggs or until the volume is doubled.
3. Then with a spatula, gently fold in the lemon zest, cinnamon and almond flour until well mixed.
4. Then pour batter on prepared pan and bake for forty minutes or until golden brown.
5. Let cool before serving.

Smoothie Bowl with Dragon Fruit

Ingredients:

- ¼ of dragon fruit, peeled and sliced
- 1 cup frozen berries
- 2 cups baby greens (mixed)
- ½ cup coconut meat

Directions:

1. Place all Ingredients in a blender and pulse until smooth.
2. Place on a bowl and allow to cool in the fridge for at least 20 minutes.
3. Garnish with whatever fruits or nuts available in your fridge.

Soothing Red Smoothie

Ingredients:

- 4 plums, pitted
- ¼ cup raspberry
- ¼ cup blueberry
- 1 tablespoon lemon juice
- 1 tablespoon linseed oil

Directions:

1. Place all Ingredients in a blender.
2. Blend until smooth.
3. Pour in a glass container and allow to chill in the fridge for at least 30 minutes.

Strawberry and Avocado Medley

Ingredients:

- 2 cups strawberry, halved
- 1 avocado, pitted and sliced
- 2 tablespoons slivered almonds

Directions:

1. Place all Ingredients in a mixing bowl.
2. Toss to combine.
3. Allow to chill in the fridge before serving.

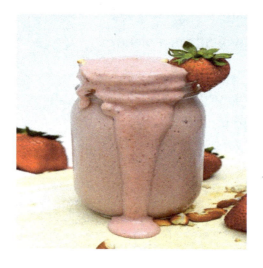

Strawberry Banana Greek Yogurt Parfaits

Ingredients:

- 1 cup plain Greek yogurt, chilled
- 1 cup pepitas
- ½ cup chopped strawberries
- ½ banana, sliced

Directions:

1. In a parfait glass, add the yogurt at the bottom of the glass.
2. Add a layer of pepitas, strawberries, and bananas.
3. Continue to layer the Ingredients until the entire glass is filled.

Summertime Fruit Salad

Ingredients:

- 1-pound strawberries, hulled and sliced thinly
- 3 medium peaches, sliced thinly
- 6 ounces blueberries
- 1 tablespoon fresh mint, chopped
- 2 tablespoons lemon juice
- 1 tablespoon honey
- 2 teaspoons balsamic vinegar

Directions:

1. In a salad bowl, combine all ingredients.
2. Gently toss to coat all ingredients.
3. Chill for at least 30 minutes before serving.

Sweet Tropical Medley Smoothie

Ingredients:

- 1 banana, peeled
- 1 sliced mango
- 1 cup fresh pineapple
- ½ cup coconut water

Directions:

1. Place all Ingredients in a blender.
2. Blend until smooth.
3. Pour in a glass container and allow to chill in the fridge for at least 30 minutes.

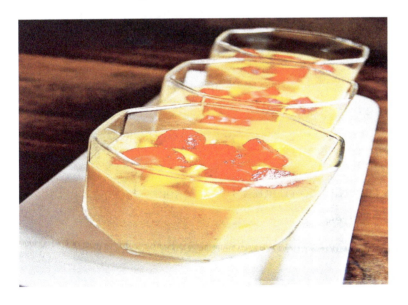

Spinach and Grilled Feta Salad

Ingredients:

- Feta cheese - 8 oz., sliced
- Black olives - 1 4 cup, sliced
- Green olives - 1 4 cup, sliced
- Baby spinach - 4 cups
- Garlic cloves - 2, minced
- Capers - 1 tsp., chopped
- Extra virgin olive oil - 2 tbsp.
- Red wine vinegar - 1 tbsp.

Directions:

1. Grill feta cheese slices over medium to high flame until brown on both sides.
2. In a salad bowl, mix green olives, black olives and spinach.
3. In a separate bowl, mix vinegar, capers and oil together to make a dressing.
4. Top salad with the dressing and cheese and it's is ready to serve.

Creamy Cool Salad

Ingredients:

- Greek yogurt - 1 2 cup
- Dill - 2 tbsp., chopped
- Lemon juice - 1 tsp.
- Cucumbers - 4, diced
- Garlic cloves - 2, minced
- Salt and pepper - to taste

Directions:

1. Mix all Ingredients in a salad bowl.
2. Add salt and pepper to suit your taste and eat.

Broccoli Salad with Caramelized Onions

Ingredients:

- Extra virgin olive oil - 3 tbsp.
- Red onions - 2, sliced
- Dried thyme - 1 tsp.
- Balsamic vinegar - 2 tbsp. vinegar
- Broccoli - 1 lb., cut into florets
- Salt and pepper - to taste

Directions:

1. Heat extra virgin olive oil in a pan over high heat and add in sliced onions. Cook for approximately 10 minutes or until the onions are caramelized. Stir in vinegar and thyme and then remove from stove.
2. Mix together the broccoli and onion mixture in a bowl, adding salt and pepper if desired. Serve and eat salad as soon as possible.

Baked Cauliflower Mixed Salad

Ingredients:

- Cauliflower - 1 lb., cut into florets
- Extra virgin olive oil - 2 tbsp.
- Dried mint - 1 tsp.
- Dried oregano - 1 tsp.
- Parsley - 2 tbsp., chopped
- Red pepper - 1, chopped
- Lemon - 1, juiced
- Green onion - 1, chopped
- Cilantro - 2 tbsp., chopped
- Salt and pepper to taste

Directions:

1. Heat oven to 350 degrees.
2. In a deep baking pan, combine olive oil, mint, cauliflower and oregano and bake for 15 minutes.
3. Once cooked, pour into a salad bowl and add remaining Ingredients:, stirring together.
4. Plate the salad and eat fresh and warm.

Quick Arugula Salad

Ingredients:

- Roasted red bell peppers - 6, sliced
- Pine nuts - 2 tbsp.
- Dried raisins - 2 tbsp.
- Red onion - 1, sliced
- Arugula - 3 cups
- Balsamic vinegar - 2 tbsp.
- Feta cheese - 4 oz., crumbled
- Extra virgin olive oil – 2 tbsp.
- Feta cheese - 4 oz., crumbled
- Salt and pepper - to taste

Directions:

1. Using a salad bowl, combine vinegar, olive oil, pine nuts, raisins, peppers and onions.
2. Add arugula and feta cheese to the mix and serve.

Bell Pepper and Tomato Salad

Ingredients:

- Roasted red bell pepper - 8, sliced
- Extra virgin olive oil - 2 tbsp.
- Chili flakes - 1 pinch
- Garlic cloves - 4, minced
- Pine nuts - 2 tbsp.
- Shallot - 1, sliced
- Cherry tomatoes - 1 cup, halved
- Parsley - 2 tbsp., chopped
- Balsamic vinegar - 1 tbsp.
- Salt and pepper - to taste

Directions:

1. Mix all Ingredients except salt and pepper in a salad bowl.
2. Season with salt and pepper if you want, to suit your taste.
3. Eat once freshly made.

One Bowl Spinach Salad

Ingredients:

- Red beets - 2, cooked and diced
- Apple cider vinegar - 1 tbsp.
- Baby spinach - 3 cups
- Greek yogurt - 1 4 cup
- Horseradish - 1 tbsp.
- Salt and pepper - to taste

Directions:

1. Mix beets and spinach in a salad bowl.
2. Add in yogurt, horseradish, and vinegar. You can also add salt and pepper if you wish.
3. Serve salad as soon as mixed.

Olive and Red Bean Salad

Ingredients:

- Red onions - 2, sliced
- Garlic cloves - 2, minced
- Balsamic vinegar - 2 tbsp.
- Green olives - 1 4 cup, sliced
- Salt and pepper - to taste
- Mixed greens - 2 cups
- Red beans - 1 can, drained
- Chili flakes - 1 pinch
- Extra virgin olive oil - 2 tbsp.
- Parsley - 2 tbsp., chopped

Directions:

1. In a salad bowl, mix all Ingredients
2. Add salt and pepper, if desired, and serve right away.

Fresh and Light Cabbage Salad

Ingredients:

- Mint - 1 tbsp., chopped
- Ground coriander - 1 2 tsp.
- Savoy cabbage - 1, shredded
- Greek yogurt - 1 2 cup
- Cumin seeds - 1 4 tsp.
- Extra virgin olive oil - 2 tbsp.
- Carrot - 1, grated
- Red onion – 1, sliced
- Honey - 1 tsp.
- Lemon zest - 1 tsp.
- Lemon juice - 2 tbsp.
- Salt and pepper - to taste

Directions:

1. In a salad bowl, mix all Ingredients
2. You can add salt and pepper to suit your taste and then mix again.
3. This salad is best when cool and freshly made.

Vegetable Patch Salad

Ingredients:

- Cauliflower - 1 bunch, cut into florets
- Zucchini - 1, sliced
- Sweet potato - 1, peeled and cubed
- Baby carrots - 1 2 lb.
- Salt and pepper - to taste
- Dried basil - 1 tsp.
- Red onions - 2, sliced
- Eggplant - 2, cubed
- Endive - 1, sliced
- Extra virgin olive oil - 3 tbsp.
- Lemon – 1, juiced
- Balsamic vinegar - 1 tbsp.

Directions:

1. Preheat oven to 350 degrees. Mix together all vegetables, basil, salt, pepper and oil in a baking dish and cook for 25 – 30 minutes.
2. After cooked, pour into salad bowl and stir in vinegar and lemon juice.
3. Dish up and serve.

Cucumber Greek yoghurt Salad

Ingredients:

- 4tbsp Greek yoghurt
- 4 large cucumbers peeled seeded and sliced
- 1 tbsp dried dill
- 1 tbsp apple cider vinegar
- 1/4 tsp garlic powder
- 1/4 tsp ground black pepper
- 1/2 tsp sugar
- 1/2 tsp salt

Directions:

1. Place all the Ingredients leaving out the cucumber into a bowl and whisk this until all is incorporated. Add your cucumber slices and toss until all is well mixed.
2. Let the salad chill 10 minutes in the refrigerator and then serve.

Chickpea Salad Recipe

Ingredients:

- Drained chickpeas: 1 can
- Halved cherry tomatoes: 1 cup
- Sun-dried chopped tomatoes: 1 2 cups
- Arugula: 2 cups
- Cubed pita bread: 1
- Pitted black olives: 1 2 cups
- 1 sliced shallot
- Cumin seeds: 1 2 teaspoon
- Coriander seeds: 1 2 teaspoon
- Chili powder: 1 4 teaspoon
- Chopped mint: 1 teaspoon
- Pepper and salt to taste
- Crumbled goat cheese: 4 oz.

Directions:

1. In a salad bowl, mix the tomatoes, chickpeas, pita bread, arugula, olives, shallot, spices and mint.
2. Stir in pepper and salt as desired to the cheese and stir.
3. You can now serve the fresh Salad.

Orange salad

Ingredients:

- 4 sliced endives
- 1 sliced red onion
- 2 oranges already cut into segments
- Extra virgin olive oil: 2 tablespoon
- Pepper and salt to taste

Directions:

1. Mix all the Ingredients in a salad bowl
2. Sprinkle pepper and salt to taste.
3. You can now serve the salad fresh.

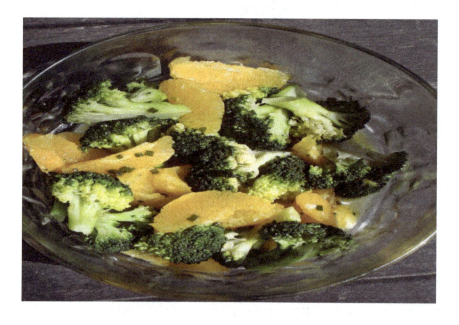

Yogurt lettuce salad recipe

Ingredients:

- Shredded Romaine lettuce: 1 head
- Sliced cucumbers: 2
- 2 minced garlic cloves
- Greek yogurt: 1 2 cup
- Dijon mustard: 1 teaspoon
- Chili powder: 1 pinch
- Extra virgin olive oil: 2 tablespoon
- Lemon juice: 1 tablespoon
- Chopped dill: 2 tablespoon
- 4 chopped mint leaves
- Pepper and salt to taste

Directions:

1. In a salad bowl, combine the lettuce with the cucumbers.
2. Add the yogurt, chili, mustard, lemon juice, dill, mint, garlic and oil in a mortar with pepper and salt as desired. Then, mix well into paste, this is the dressing for the salad .
3. Top the Salad with the dressing then serve fresh.

Fruit de salad recipe

Ingredients:

- Cubed seedless watermelon: 8 oz.
- Halved red grapes: 4 oz.
- 2 Sliced cucumbers
- Halved strawberries: 1 cup
- Cubed feta cheese: 6 oz.
- Balsamic vinegar: 2 tablespoon
- Arugula: 2 cups

Directions:

1. In a salad bowl, mix the strawberries, grapes, arugula, cucumbers, feta cheese and watermelon together.
2. Top the salad with vinegar and serve fresh.

Chickpea with mint salad recipe

Ingredients:

- 1 diced cucumber
- Sliced black olives: 1 4 cup
- Chopped mint: 2 tablespoon
- Cooked and drained short pasta: 4 oz.
- Arugula: 2 cups
- Drained chickpeas: 1 can
- 1 sliced shallot
- Chopped Parsley: 1 2 cup
- Halved cherry tomatoes: 1 2 pound
- Sliced green olives: 1 4 cup
- 1 juiced lemon
- Extra virgin olive oil: 2 tablespoon
- Chopped walnut: 1 2 cup
- Pepper and salt to taste

Directions:

1. Mix the chickpeas with the other Ingredients in a salad bowl
2. Top with oil and lemon juice, sprinkle pepper and salt then mix well.
3. Refrigerate the Salad (can last in a sealed container for about 2 days) or serve fresh.

Grapy Fennel salad

Ingredients:

- Grape seed oil: 1 tablespoon
- Chopped dill: 1 tablespoon
- 1 finely sliced fennel bulb
- Toasted almond slices: 2 tablespoon
- Chopped mint: 1 teaspoon
- 1 grapefruit already cut into segments
- 1 orange already cut into segments
- Pepper and salt as desired

Directions:

1. Using a platter, mix the grapefruit and orange segments with the fennel bulb
2. Add the mint, almond slices and dill, top with the oil and add pepper and salt as desired.
3. You can now serve the Salad fresh.

Greenie salad recipe

Ingredients:

- Extra virgin olive oil: 2 tablespoon
- Mixed greens: 12 oz.
- Pitted black olives: 1 2 cup
- Pitted green olives: 1 4 cup
- Sherry vinegar: 2 tablespoon
- Pitted Kalamata olives: 1 2 cup
- Almond slices: 2 tablespoon
- Parmesan shavings: 2 oz.
- Sliced Parma ham: 2 oz.
- Pepper and salt as desired

Directions:

1. Stir the almonds, olives and mixed greens together in a salad bowl
2. Drizzle the oil and vinegar then sprinkle pepper and salt as you want.
3. Top with the Parma ham and Parmesan shavings before serving.
4. You can now serve fresh.

A Refreshing Detox Salad

Ingredients:

- 1 large apple, diced
- 1 large beet, coarsely grated
- 1 large carrot, coarsely grated
- 1 tbsp chia seeds
- 2 tbsp almonds, chopped
- 2 tbsp lemon juice
- 2 tbsp pumpkin seed oil
- 4 cups mixed greens

Directions:

1. In a medium salad bowl, except for mixed greens, combine all ingredients thoroughly.
2. Into 4 salad plates, divide the mixed greens.
3. Evenly top mixed greens with the salad bowl mixture.
4. Serve and enjoy.

Amazingly Fresh Carrot Salad

Ingredients:

- ¼ tsp chipotle powder
- 1 bunch scallions, sliced
- 1 cup cherry tomatoes, halved
- 1 large avocado, diced
- 1 tbsp chili powder
- 1 tbsp lemon juice
- 2 tbsp olive oil
- 3 tbsp lime juice
- 4 cups carrots, spiralized
- salt to taste

Directions:

1. In a salad bowl, mix and arrange avocado, cherry tomatoes, scallions and spiralized carrots. Set aside.
2. In a small bowl, whisk salt, chipotle powder, chili powder, olive oil, lemon juice and lime juice thoroughly.
3. Pour dressing over noodle salad. Toss to coat well.
4. Serve and enjoy at room temperature.

Anchovy and Orange Salad

Ingredients:

- 1 small red onion, sliced into thin rounds
- 1 tbsp fresh lemon juice
- 1/8 tsp pepper or more to taste
- 16 oil cure Kalamata olives
- 2 tsp finely minced fennel fronds for garnish
- 3 tbsp extra virgin olive oil
- 4 small oranges, preferably blood oranges
- 6 anchovy fillets

Directions:

1. With a paring knife, peel oranges including the membrane that surrounds it.
2. In a plate, slice oranges into thin circles and allow plate to catch the orange juices.
3. On serving plate, arrange orange slices on a layer.
4. Sprinkle oranges with onion, followed by olives and then anchovy fillets.
5. Drizzle with oil, lemon juice and orange juice.
6. Sprinkle with pepper.

7. Allow salad to stand for 30 minutes at room temperature to allow the flavors to develop.
8. To serve, garnish with fennel fronds and enjoy.

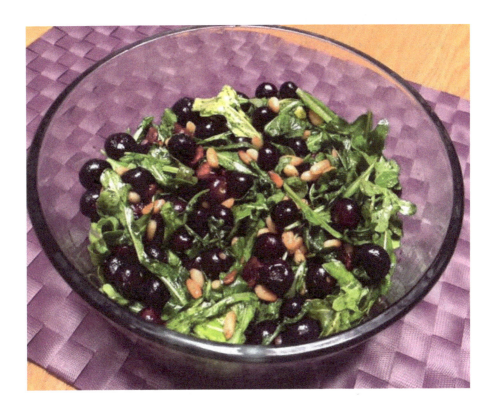

Arugula with Blueberries 'n Almonds

Ingredients:

- ½ cup slivered almonds
- ½ cup blueberries, fresh
- 1 ripe red pear, sliced
- 1 shallot, minced
- 1 tsp minced garlic
- 1 tsp whole grain mustard
- 2 tbsp fresh lemon juice
- 3 tbsp extra virgin olive oil
- 6 cups arugula

Directions:

1. In a big mixing bowl, mix garlic, olive oil, lemon juice and mustard.
2. Once thoroughly mixed, add remaining ingredients.
3. Toss to coat.
4. Equally divide into two bowls, serve and enjoy.

Asian Peanut Sauce Over Noodle Salad

Ingredients:

- 1 cup shredded green cabbage
- 1 cup shredded red cabbage
- 1/4 cup chopped cilantro
- 1/4 cup chopped peanuts
- 1/4 cup chopped scallions
- 4 cups shiritake noodles (drained and rinsed)
- Asian Peanut Sauce Ingredients
- ¼ cup sugar free peanut butter
- ¼ teaspoon cayenne pepper
- ½ cup filtered water
- ½ teaspoon kosher salt
- 1 tablespoon fish sauce (or coconut aminos for vegan)
- 1 tablespoon granulated erythritol sweetener
- 1 tablespoon lime juice
- 1 tablespoon toasted sesame oil
- 1 tablespoon wheat-free soy sauce
- 1 teaspoon minced garlic
- 2 tablespoons minced ginger

Directions:

1. In a large salad bowl, combine all noodle salad ingredients and toss well to mix.
2. In a blender, mix all sauce ingredients and pulse until smooth and creamy.
3. Pour sauce over the salad and toss well to coat.
4. Evenly divide into four equal servings and enjoy.

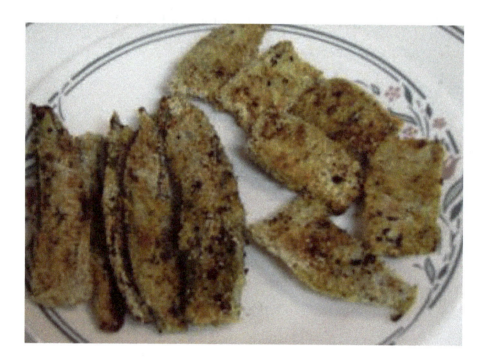

Vegetable Fritters

Ingredients:

- Egg (3, beaten)
- Milk (8 Fl oz)
- Whole wheat flour (8 oz)
- Baking powder (1 tbsp)
- Salt (½ tsp)
- Maple syrup (1/2 oz)

<u>Vegetables:</u>

- Carrot (12 oz,)
- Baby lima beans (12 oz)
- Asparagus (12 oz)
- Celery (12 oz)
- Turnip (12 oz)
- Eggplant (12 oz)
- Cauliflower (12 oz)
- Zucchini (12 oz)
- Parsnips (12 oz)

Directions:

1. Combine the eggs and milk.
2. Mix the flour, baking powder, salt, and maple syrup. Add to the milk and eggs and mix until smooth.

3. Let the batter stand for several hours in a refrigerator.
4. Stir the cold, cooked vegetable into the batter.
5. Drop with a No. 24 scoop into deep fat at 350 F. Toss the content from the scoop carefully in the hot oil. Fry until golden brown.
6. Drain well and serve.

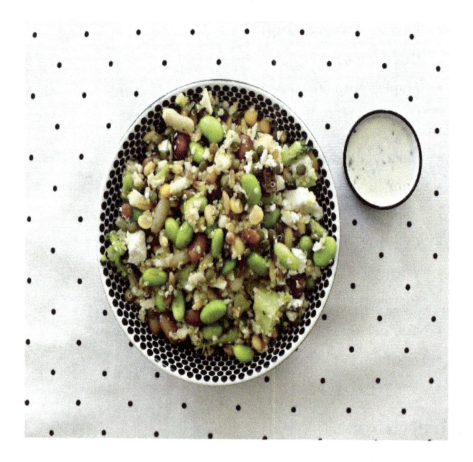

Asian Salad with pistachios

Ingredients:

- ¼ cup chopped pistachios
- ¼ cup green onions, sliced
- 1 bunch watercress, trimmed
- 1 cup red bell pepper, diced
- 2 cups medium sized fennel bulb, thinly sliced
- 2 tbsp vegetable oil
- 3 cups Asian pears, cut into matchstick size
- 3 tbsp fresh lime juice

Directions

1. In a large salad bowl, mix pistachios, green onions, bell pepper, fennel, watercress and pears.
2. In a small bowl, mix vegetable oil and lime juice. Season with pepper and salt to taste.
3. Pour dressing to salad and gently mix before serving.

Balela Salad from the Middle East

Ingredients:

- 1 jalapeno, finely chopped (optional)
- 1/2 green bell pepper, cored and chopped
- 2 1/2 cups grape tomatoes, slice in halves
- 1/2 cup sun-dried tomatoes
- 1/2 cup freshly chopped parsley leaves
- 1/2 cup freshly chopped mint or basil leaves
- 1/3 cup pitted Kalamata olives
- 1/4 cup pitted green olives
- 3 1/2 cups cooked chickpeas, drained and rinsed
- 3–5 green onions, both white and green parts, chopped

Dressing Ingredients

- 1 garlic clove, minced
- 1 tsp ground sumac
- 1/2 tsp Aleppo pepper
- 1/4 cup Early Harvest Greek extra virgin olive oil
- 1/4 to 1/2 tsp crushed red pepper (optional)
- 2 tbsp lemon juice
- 2 tbsp white wine vinegar
- Salt and black pepper, a generous pinch to your taste

Directions:

1. Mix together the salad ingredients in a large salad bowl.
2. In a separate smaller bowl or jar, mix together the dressing ingredients.
3. Drizzle the dressing over the salad and gently toss to coat.
4. Set aside for 30 minutes to allow the flavors to mix.
5. Serve and enjoy.

Blue Cheese and Portobello Salad

Ingredients:

- ½ cup croutons
- 1 tbsp merlot wine
- 1 tbsp water
- 1 tsp minced garlic
- 1 tsp olive oil
- 2 large Portobello mushrooms, stemmed, wiped clean and cut into
- bite sized pieces
- 2 pieces roasted red peppers (canned), sliced
- 2 tbsp balsamic vinegar
- 2 tbsp crumbled blue cheese
- 4 slices red onion
- 6 asparagus stalks cut into 1-inch sections
- 6 cups Bibb lettuce, chopped
- Ground pepper to taste

Directions:

1. On medium fire, place a small pan and heat oil. Once hot, add onions and mushrooms. For 4 to 6 minutes, sauté until tender.

2. Add garlic and for a minute continue sautéing.
3. Pour in wine and cook for a minute.
4. Bring an inch of water to a boil in a pot with steamer basket. Once boiling, add asparagus, steam for two to three minutes or until crisp and tender, while covered. Once cooked, remove basket from pot and set aside.
5. In a small bowl whisk thoroughly black pepper, water, balsamic vinegar, and blue cheese.
6. To serve, place 3 cups of lettuce on each plate. Add 1 roasted pepper, ½ of asparagus, ½ of mushroom mixture, whisk blue cheese dressing before drizzling equally on to plates. Garnish with croutons, serve and enjoy.

Blue Cheese and Arugula Salad

Ingredients:

- ¼ cup crumbled blue cheese
- 1 tsp Dijon mustard
- 1-pint fresh figs, quartered
- 2 bags arugula
- 3 tbsp Balsamic Vinegar
- 3 tbsp olive oil
- Pepper and salt to taste

Directions:

1. Whisk thoroughly together pepper, salt, olive oil, Dijon mustard, and balsamic vinegar to make the dressing. Set aside in the ref for at least 30 minutes to marinate and allow the spices to combine.
2. On four serving plates, evenly arrange arugula and top with blue cheese and figs.
3. Drizzle each plate of salad with 1 ½ tbsp of prepared dressing.
4. Serve and enjoy.

Broccoli Salad Moroccan Style

Ingredients:

- ¼ tsp sea salt
- ¼ tsp ground cinnamon
- ½ tsp ground turmeric
- ¾ tsp ground ginger
- ½ tbsp extra virgin olive oil
- ½ tbsp apple cider vinegar
- 2 tbsp chopped green onion
- 1/3 cup coconut cream
- ½ cup carrots, shredded
- 1 small head of broccoli, chopped

Directions:

1. In a large salad bowl, mix well salt, cinnamon, turmeric, ginger, olive oil, and vinegar.
2. Add remaining ingredients, tossing well to coat.
3. Pop in the ref for at least 30 to 60 minutes before serving.

Classic Greek Salad

Ingredients:

- ¼ cup extra virgin olive oil, plus more for drizzling
- ¼ cup red wine vinegar
- 1 4-oz block Greek feta cheese packed in brine
- 1 cup Kalamata olives, halved and pitted
- 1 lemon, juiced and zested
- 1 small red onion, halved and thinly sliced
- 1 tsp dried oregano
- 1 tsp honey
- 14 small vine-ripened tomatoes, quartered
- 5 Persian cucumbers
- Fresh oregano leaves for topping, optional
- Pepper to taste
- Salt to taste

Directions:

1. In a bowl of ice water, soak red onions with 2 tbsp salt.
2. In a large bowl, whisk well ¼ tsp pepper, ½ tsp salt, dried oregano, honey, lemon zest, lemon juice, and vinegar. Slowly pour olive oil in a steady stream as you

briskly whisk mixture. Continue whisking until emulsified.
3. Add olives and tomatoes, toss to coat with dressing.
4. Alternatingly peel cucumber leaving strips of skin on. Trim ends slice lengthwise and chop in ½-inch thick cubes. Add into bowl of tomatoes.
5. Drain onions and add into bowl of tomatoes. Toss well to coat and mix.
6. Drain feta and slice into four equal rectangles.
7. Divide Greek salad into serving plates, top each with oregano and feta.
8. To serve, season with pepper and drizzle with oil and enjoy.

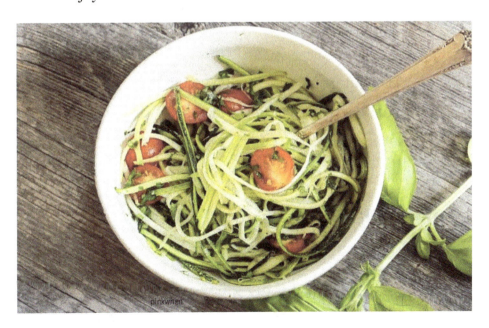

Cold Zucchini Noodle Bowl

Ingredients:

- ¼ cup basil leaves, roughly chopped
- ¼ cup olive oil
- ¼ tsp sea salt
- ½ tsp salt1 tsp garlic powder
- 1 lb. peeled and uncooked shrimp
- 1 tsp lemon zest
- 1 tsp lime zest
- 2 tbsp butter
- 2 tbsp lemon juice
- 2 tbsp lime juice
- 3 clementine, peeled and separated
- 4 cups zucchini, spirals or noodles
- pinch of black pepper

Directions:

1. Make zucchini noodles and set aside.
2. On medium fire, place a large nonstick saucepan and heat butter.

3. Meanwhile, pat dry shrimps and season with salt and garlic. Add into hot saucepan and sauté for 6 minutes or until opaque and cooked.
4. Remove from pan, transfer to a bowl and put aside.
5. Right away, add zucchini noodles to still hot pan and stir fry for a minute. Leave noodles on pan as you prepare the dressing.
6. Blend well salt, olive oil, juice and zest in a small bowl.
7. Then place noodles into salad bowl, top with shrimp, pour oil mixture, basil and clementine. Toss to mix well.
8. Refrigerate for an hour before serving.

Coleslaw Asian Style

Ingredients:

- ½ cup chopped fresh cilantro
- 1 ½ tbsp minced garlic
- 2 carrots, julienned
- 2 cups shredded napa cabbage
- 2 cups thinly sliced red cabbage
- 2 red bell peppers, thinly sliced
- 2 tbsp minced fresh ginger root
- 3 tbsp brown sugar
- 3 tbsp soy sauce
- 5 cups thinly sliced green cabbage
- 5 tbsp creamy peanut butter
- 6 green onions, chopped
- 6 tbsp rice wine vinegar
- 6 tbsp vegetable oil

Directions:

1. Mix thoroughly the following in a medium bowl: garlic, ginger, brown sugar, soy sauce, peanut butter, oil and rice vinegar.
2. In a separate bowl, blend well cilantro, green onions, carrots, bell pepper, Napa cabbage, red cabbage and

green cabbage. Pour in the peanut sauce above and toss to mix well.

3. Serve and enjoy.

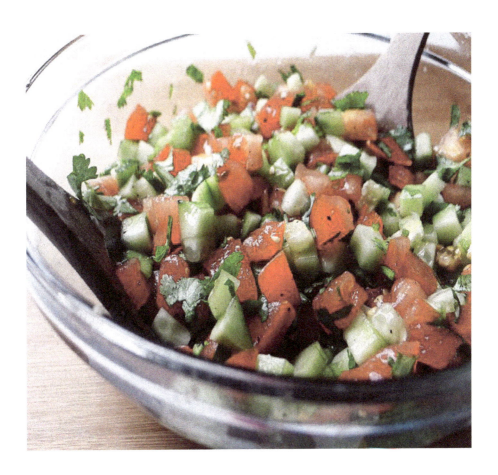

Cucumber and Tomato Salad

Ingredients:

- Ground pepper to taste
- Salt to taste
- 1 tbsp fresh lemon juice
- 1 onion, chopped
- 1 cucumber, peeled and diced
- 2 tomatoes, chopped
- 4 cups spinach

Directions:

1. In a salad bowl, mix onions, cucumbers and tomatoes.
2. Season with pepper and salt to taste.
3. Add lemon juice and mix well.
4. Add spinach, toss to coat, serve and enjoy.

Cucumber Salad Japanese Style

Ingredients:

- 1 ½ tsp minced fresh ginger root
- 1 tsp salt
- 1/3 cup rice vinegar
- 2 large cucumbers, ribbon cut
- 4 tsp white sugar

Directions:

1. Mix well ginger, salt, sugar and vinegar in a small bowl.
2. Add ribbon cut cucumbers and mix well.
3. Let stand for at least one hour in the ref before serving.

Easy Garden Salad with Arugula

Ingredients:

- ¼ cup grated parmesan cheese
- ¼ cup pine nuts
- 1 cup cherry tomatoes, halved
- 1 large avocado, sliced into ½ inch cubes
- 1 tbsp rice vinegar
- 2 tbsp olive oil or grapeseed oil
- 4 cups young arugula leaves, rinsed and dried
- Black pepper, freshly ground
- Salt to taste

Directions:

1. Get a bowl with cover, big enough to hold the salad and mix together the parmesan cheese, vinegar, oil, pine nuts, cherry tomatoes and arugula.
2. Season with pepper and salt according to how you like it. Place the lid and jiggle the covered bowl to combine the salad.
3. Serve the salad topped with sliced avocadoes.

Easy Quinoa & Pear Salad

Ingredients:

- ¼ cup chopped parsley
- ¼ cup chopped scallions
- ¼ cup lime juice
- ¼ cup red onion, diced
- ½ cup diced carrots
- ½ cup diced celery
- ½ cup diced cucumber
- ½ cup diced red pepper
- ½ cup dried wild blueberries
- ½ cup olive oil
- ½ cup spicy pecans, chopped
- 1 tbsp chopped parsley
- 1 tsp honey
- 1 tsp sea salt
- 2 fresh pears, cut into chunks
- 3 cups cooked quinoa

Directions:

1. In a small bowl mix well olive oil, salt, lime juice, honey, and parsley. Set aside.
2. In large salad bowl, add remaining ingredients and toss to mix well.

3. Pour dressing and toss well to coat.
4. Serve and enjoy.

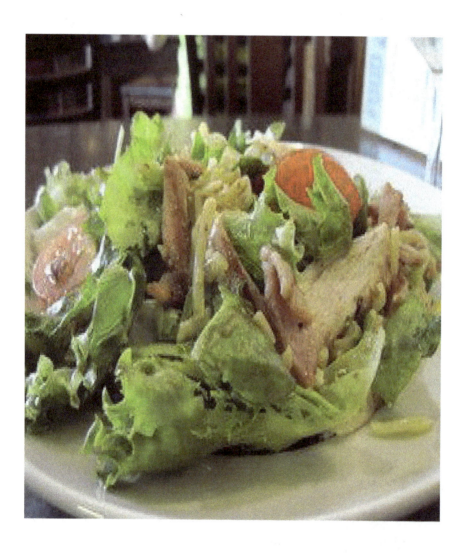

Easy-Peasy Club Salad

Ingredients:

- ½ cup cherry tomatoes, halved
- ½ teaspoon garlic powder
- ½ teaspoon onion powder
- 1 cup diced cucumber
- 1 tablespoon Dijon mustard
- 1 tablespoon milk
- 1 teaspoon dried parsley
- 2 tablespoons mayonnaise
- 2 tablespoons sour cream
- 3 cups romaine lettuce, torn into pieces
- 3 large hard-boiled eggs, sliced
- 4 ounces cheddar cheese, cubed

Directions:

1. Make the dressing by mixing garlic powder, onion powder, dried parsley, mayonnaise, and sour cream in a small bowl.
2. Add a tablespoon of milk and mix well. If you want the dressing thinner, you can add more milk.
3. In a salad platter, layer salad ingredients with Dijon mustard in the middle.
4. Evenly drizzle with dressing and toss well to coat.

Fennel and Seared Scallops Salad

Ingredients:

- ¼ tsp salt
- ½ large fennel bulb, halved, cored and very thinly sliced
- ½ tsp whole fennel seeds, freshly ground
- 1 large pink grapefruit
- 1 lb. fresh sea scallops, muscle removed, room temperature
- 1 tbsp olive oil, divided
- 1 tsp raw honey
- 12 whole almonds chopped coarsely and lightly toasted
- 4 cups red leaf lettuce, cored and torn into bite sized pieces
- A pinch of ground pepper

Directions:

1. To catch the juices, work over a bowl. Peel and segment grapefruit. Strain the juice in a cup.
2. For the dressing, whisk together in a small bowl black pepper, 1/8 tsp salt, 1/8 tsp ground fennel, honey, 2 tsp

water, 2 tsp oil and 3 tbsp of pomegranate juice. Set aside 1 tbsp of the dressing.
3. Pat scallops dry with a paper towel and season with remaining salt and ½ tsp ground fennel.
4. On medium fire, place a nonstick skillet and brush with 1 tsp oil. Once heated, add ½ of scallops and cook until lightly browned or for 5 minutes each side. Transfer to a plate and keep warm as you cook the second batch using the same process.
5. Mix together dressing, lettuce and fennel in a large salad bowl. Divide evenly onto 4 salad plates.
6. Evenly top each salad with scallops, grapefruit segments and almonds. Drizzle with reserved dressing, serve and enjoy.

Fruity Asparagus-Quinoa Salad

Ingredients:

- ¼ cup chopped pecans, toasted
- ½ cup finely chopped white onion
- ½ jalapeno pepper, diced
- ½ lb. asparagus, sliced to 2-inch lengths, steamed and chilled
- ½ tsp kosher salt
- 1 cup fresh orange sections
- 1 cup uncooked quinoa
- 1 tsp olive oil
- 2 cups water
- 2 tbsp minced red onion
- 5 dates, pitted and chopped

<u>Dressing ingredients</u>
- ¼ tsp ground black pepper
- ¼ tsp kosher salt
- 1 garlic clove, minced
- 1 tbsp olive oil
- 2 tbsp chopped fresh mint
- 2 tbsp fresh lemon juice
- Mint sprigs – optional

Directions:

1. Wash and rub with your hands the quinoa in a bowl at least three times, discarding water each and every time.
2. On medium high fire, place a large nonstick fry pan and heat 1 tsp olive oil. For two minutes, sauté onions before adding quinoa and sautéing for another five minutes.
3. Add ½ tsp salt and 2 cups water and bring to a boil. Lower fire to a simmer, cover and cook for 15 minutes. Turn off fire and let stand until water is absorbed.
4. Add pepper, asparagus, dates, pecans and orange sections into a salad bowl. Add cooked quinoa, toss to mix well.
5. In a small bowl, whisk mint, garlic, black pepper, salt, olive oil and lemon juice to create the dressing.
6. Pour dressing over salad, serve and enjoy.

Garden Salad with Balsamic Vinegar

Ingredients:

- 1 cup baby arugula
- 1 cup spinach
- 1 tbsp raisins
- 1 tbsp almonds, shaved or chopped
- 1 tbsp balsamic vinegar
- ½ tbsp extra virgin olive oil

Directions:

1. In a plate, mix arugula and spinach.
2. Top with raisins and almonds.
3. Drizzle olive oil and balsamic vinegar.
4. Serve and enjoy.

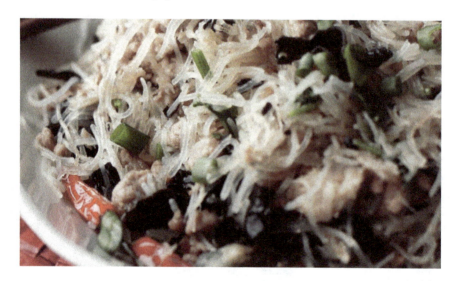

Rice with Vermicelli

Ingredients:

- 2 cups short-grain rice
- 3½ cups water
- ¼ cup olive oil
- 1 cup broken vermicelli pasta
- Salt

Directions:

1. Rinse the rice under cold water until the water runs clean. Place the rice in a bowl, cover with water, and let soak for 10 minutes. Drain and set aside.
2. In a medium pot over medium heat, heat the olive oil.
3. Stir in the vermicelli and cook for 2 to 3 minutes, stirring continuously, until golden.
4. Add the rice and cook for 1 minute, stirring, so the rice is well coated in the oil.
5. Add the water and a pinch of salt and bring the liquid to a boil. Reduce the heat to low, cover the pot, and simmer for 20 minutes.
6. Remove from the heat and let rest, covered, for 10 minutes. Fluff with a fork and serve.

Fava Beans and Rice

Ingredients:

- ¼ cup olive oil
- 4 cups fresh fava beans
- 4½ cups water
- 2 cups basmati rice
- 1/8 teaspoon salt
- 1/8 teaspoon black pepper
- 2 tablespoons pine nuts, toasted
- ½ cup chopped fresh garlic chives

Directions:

1. In a large saucepan over medium heat, heat the olive oil.
2. Add the fava beans and drizzle them with a bit of water. Cook for 10 minutes.
3. Gently stir in the rice. Add the water, salt, and pepper. Increase the heat and bring the mixture to a boil. Cover, reduce the heat to low, and simmer for 15 minutes.
4. Turn off the heat and let the mixture rest for 10 minutes before serving. Sprinkle with toasted pine nuts and chives.

Buttered Fava Beans

Ingredients:

- ½ cup vegetable broth
- 4 pounds fava beans
- ¼ cup fresh tarragon
- 1 teaspoon chopped fresh thyme
- ¼ teaspoon black pepper
- 1/8 teaspoon salt
- 2 tablespoons butter
- 1 garlic clove, minced
- 2 tablespoons chopped fresh parsley

Directions:

1. In a shallow pan over medium heat, bring the vegetable broth to a boil.
2. Add the fava beans, 2 tablespoons of tarragon, the thyme, pepper, and salt. Cook for 10 minutes.
3. Stir in the butter, garlic, and remaining 2 tablespoons of tarragon. Cook for 2 to 3 minutes.
4. Sprinkle with the parsley.

Freekeh

Ingredients:

- 4 tablespoons Ghee
- 1 onion, chopped
- 3½ cups vegetable broth
- 1 teaspoon ground allspice
- 2 cups freekeh
- 2 tablespoons pine nuts

Directions:

1. In a heavy-bottomed saucepan over medium heat, melt the ghee.
2. Stir in the onion and cook for about 5 minutes, stirring constantly, until the onion is golden.
3. Pour in the vegetable broth, add the allspice, and bring to a boil.
4. Stir in the freekeh and return the mixture to a boil. Reduce the heat to low, cover the pan, and simmer for 30 minutes, stirring occasionally.
5. Spoon the freekeh into a serving dish and top with the toasted pine nuts.

Fried Rice Balls with Tomato Sauce

Ingredients:

- 1 cup bread crumbs
- 2 cups cooked risotto
- 2 large eggs, divided
- ¼ cup freshly grated Parmesan cheese
- 8 fresh baby mozzarella balls
- 2 tablespoons water
- 1 cup corn oil
- 1 cup Basic Tomato Basil Sauce

Directions:

1. Pour the bread crumbs into a small bowl and set aside.
2. In a medium bowl, stir together the risotto, 1 egg, and the Parmesan cheese until well combined.
3. Moisten your hands with a little water to prevent sticking and divide the risotto mixture into 8 pieces. Place them on a clean work surface and flatten each piece.
4. Place 1 mozzarella ball on each flattened rice disk. Close the rice around the mozzarella to form a ball. Repeat until you finish all the balls.

5. In the same medium, now-empty bowl, whisk the remaining egg and the water.
6. Dip each prepared risotto ball into the egg wash and roll it in the bread crumbs. Set aside.
7. In a large sauté pan or skillet over high heat, heat the corn oil for about 3 minutes.
8. Gently lower the risotto balls into the hot oil and fry for 5 to 8 minutes until golden brown. Stir them, as needed, to ensure the entire surface is fried. Using a slotted spoon, transfer the fried balls to paper towels to drain.
9. In a medium saucepan over medium heat, heat the tomato sauce for 5 minutes, stirring occasionally, and serve the warm sauce alongside the rice balls.

Spanish-Style Rice

Ingredients:

- ¼ cup olive oil
- 1 small onion
- 1 red bell pepper
- 1½ cups white rice
- 1 teaspoon sweet paprika
- ½ teaspoon ground cumin
- ½ teaspoon ground coriander
- 1 garlic clove, minced
- 3 tablespoons tomato paste
- 3 cups vegetable broth
- 1/8 teaspoon salt

Directions:

1. In a large heavy-bottomed skillet over medium heat, heat the olive oil.
2. Stir in the onion and red bell pepper. Cook for 5 minutes or until softened.
3. Add the rice, paprika, cumin, and coriander and cook for 2 minutes, stirring often.
4. Add the garlic, tomato paste, vegetable broth, and salt. Stir to combine, taste, and season with more salt, as needed.

5. Increase the heat to bring the mixture to a boil. Reduce the heat to low, cover the skillet, and simmer for 20 minutes.
6. Let the rice rest, covered, for 5 minutes before serving.

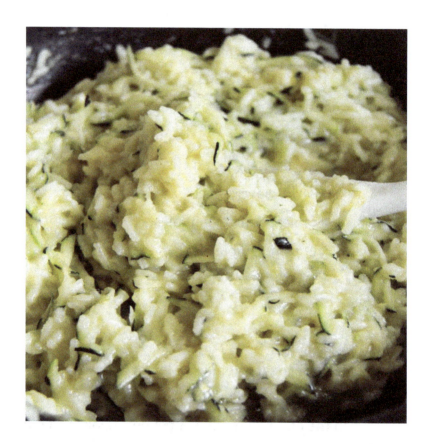

Zucchini with Rice and Tzatziki

Ingredients:

- ¼ cup olive oil
- 1 onion
- 3 zucchinis
- 1 cup vegetable broth
- ½ cup chopped fresh dill
- 1 cup short-grain rice
- 2 tablespoons pine nuts
- 1 cup Tzatziki Sauce, Plain Yogurt

Directions:

1. In a heavy-bottomed pot over medium heat, heat the olive oil.
2. Add the onion, turn the heat to medium-low, and sauté for 5 minutes.
3. Add the zucchini and cook for 2 minutes more.
4. Stir in the vegetable broth and dill and season with salt and pepper. Increase the heat to medium and bring the mixture to a boil.

5. Stir in the rice and let it boil. Set to very low heat, cover the pot, and cook for 15 minutes. Remove from the heat and let the rice rest, covered, for 10 minutes.
6. Spoon the rice onto a serving platter, sprinkle with the pine nuts, and serve with tzatziki sauce.

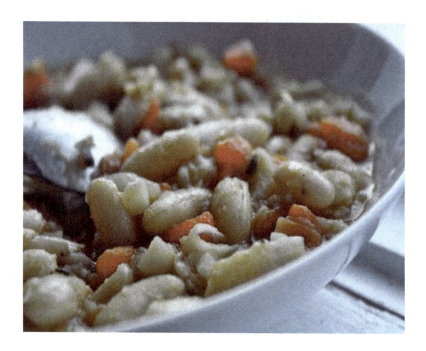

Cannellini Beans with Rosemary and Garlic Aioli

Ingredients:

- 4 cups cooked cannellini beans
- 4 cups water
- ½ teaspoon salt
- 3 tablespoons olive oil
- 2 tablespoons chopped fresh rosemary
- ½ cup Garlic Aioli
- ¼ teaspoon freshly ground black pepper

Directions:

1. In a medium saucepan over medium heat, combine the cannellini beans, water, and salt. Bring to a boil. Cook for 5 minutes. Drain.
2. In a skillet over medium heat, heat the olive oil.
3. Add the beans. Stir in the rosemary and aioli. Reduce the heat to medium-low and cook, stirring, just to heat through. Season with pepper and serve.

Jeweled Rice

Ingredients:

- ½ cup olive oil, divided
- 1 onion, finely chopped
- 1 garlic clove, minced
- ½ teaspoon fresh ginger
- 4½ cups water
- 1 teaspoon salt
- 1 teaspoon ground turmeric
- 2 cups basmati rice
- 1 cup fresh sweet peas
- 2 carrots
- ½ cup dried cranberries
- Grated zest of 1 orange
- 1/8 teaspoon cayenne pepper
- ¼ cup slivered almonds

Directions:

1. In a large heavy-bottomed pot over medium heat, heat ¼ cup of olive oil.
2. Add the onion and cook for 4 minutes. Add the garlic and ginger and cook for 1 minute more.

3. Stir in the water, ¾ teaspoon of salt, and the turmeric. Bring the mixture to a boil. Mix in the rice and boil. Select heat to low, cover the pot, and cook for 15 minutes. Turn off the heat. Let the rice rest on the burner, covered, for 10 minutes.
4. Meanwhile, in a medium sauté pan or skillet over medium-low heat, heat the remaining ¼ cup of olive oil. Stir in the peas and carrots. Cook for 5 minutes.
5. Stir in the cranberries and orange zest. Season with the remaining ¼ teaspoon of salt and the cayenne. Cook for 1 to 2 minutes.
6. Spoon the rice onto a serving platter. Top with the peas and carrots and sprinkle with the toasted almonds.

Asparagus Risotto

Ingredients:

- 5 cups vegetable broth
- 3 tablespoons unsalted butter
- 1 tablespoon olive oil
- 1 small onion, chopped
- 1½ cups Arborio rice
- 1-pound fresh asparagus
- ¼ cup freshly grated Parmesan cheese, plus more for serving

Directions:

1. In a saucepan over medium heat, bring the vegetable broth to a boil. Turn the heat to low and keep the broth at a steady simmer.
2. In a 4-quart heavy-bottomed saucepan over medium heat, melt 2 tablespoons of butter with the olive oil. Add the onion and cook for 2 to 3 minutes.
3. Add the rice and stir with a wooden spoon while cooking for 1 minute until the grains are well coated in the butter and oil.

4. Stir in ½ cup of warm broth. Cook, stirring often, for about 5 minutes until the broth is completely absorbed.
5. Add the asparagus stalks and another ½ cup of broth. Cook, stirring often, until the liquid is absorbed. Continue adding the broth, ½ cup at a time, and cooking until it is completely absorbed before adding the next ½ cup. Stir frequently to prevent sticking. After about 20 minutes, the rice should be cooked but still firm.
6. Add the asparagus tips, the remaining 1 tablespoon of butter, and the Parmesan cheese. Stir vigorously to combine.
7. Remove from the heat, top with additional Parmesan cheese, if desired, and serve immediately.

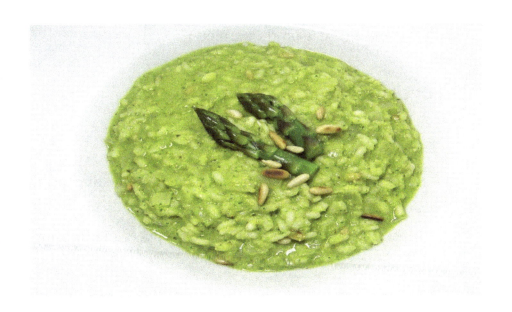

Vegetable Paella

Ingredients:

- ¼ cup olive oil
- 1 large sweet onion
- 1 large red bell pepper
- 1 large green bell pepper
- 3 garlic cloves
- 1 teaspoon smoked paprika
- 5 saffron threads
- 1 zucchini, cut into ½-inch cubes
- 4 large ripe tomatoes
- 1½ cups short-grain Spanish rice
- 3 cups vegetable broth, warmed

Directions:

1. Preheat the oven to 350°F.
2. In a paella pan or large oven-safe skillet over medium heat, heat the olive oil.
3. Add the onion and red and green bell peppers and cook for 10 minutes.

4. Stir in the garlic, paprika, saffron threads, zucchini, and tomatoes. Turn the heat to medium-low and cook for 10 minutes.
5. Stir in the rice and vegetable broth. Increase the heat to bring the paella to a boil. Reduce the heat to medium-low and cook for 15 minutes. Cover the pan with aluminum foil and put it in the oven.
6. Bake for 10 minutes or until the broth is absorbed.

Eggplant and Rice Casserole

Ingredients:

<ins>For sauce</ins>
- ½ cup olive oil
- 1 small onion
- 4 garlic cloves
- 6 ripe tomatoes
- 2 tablespoons tomato paste
- 1 teaspoon dried oregano
- ¼ teaspoon ground nutmeg
- ¼ teaspoon ground cumin

<ins>For casserole</ins>
- 4 (6-inch) Japanese eggplants
- 2 tablespoons olive oil
- 1 cup cooked rice
- 2 tablespoons pine nuts
- 1 cup water

Directions:

<ins>For sauce</ins>
1. In a heavy-bottomed saucepan over medium heat, heat the olive oil. Add the onion and cook for 5 minutes.

2. Stir in the garlic, tomatoes, tomato paste, oregano, nutmeg, and cumin. Bring to a boil. Cover, reduce heat to low, and simmer for
3. 10 minutes. Remove and set aside.

<u>For casserole</u>
1. Preheat the broiler.
2. While the sauce simmers, drizzle the eggplant with the olive oil and place them on a baking sheet. Broil for about 5 minutes until golden. Remove and let cool.
3. Turn the oven to 375°F. Arrange the cooled eggplant, cut-side up, in a 9-by-13-inch baking dish. Gently scoop out some flesh to make room for the stuffing.
4. In a bowl, combine half the tomato sauce, the cooked rice, and pine nuts. Fill each eggplant half with the rice mixture.
5. In the same bowl, combine the remaining tomato sauce and water. Pour over the eggplant.
6. Bake, covered, for 20 minutes.

Many Vegetable Couscous

Ingredients:

- ¼ cup olive oil
- 1 onion, chopped
- 4 garlic cloves, minced
- 2 jalapeño peppers
- ½ teaspoon ground cumin
- ½ teaspoon ground coriander
- 1 (28-ounce) can crushed tomatoes
- 2 tablespoons tomato paste
- 1/8 teaspoon salt
- 2 bay leaves
- 11 cups water, divided
- 4 carrots, peeled and cut into 2-inch pieces
- 2 zucchinis
- 1 acorn squash
- 1 (15-ounce) can chickpeas
- ¼ cup chopped Preserved Lemons (optional)
- 3 cups couscous

Directions:

1. In a large heavy-bottomed pot over medium heat, heat the olive oil. Stir in the onion and cook for 4 minutes. Stir in the garlic, jalapeños, cumin, and coriander. Cook for 1 minute.
2. Add the tomatoes, tomato paste, salt, bay leaves, and 8 cups of water. Bring the mixture to a boil.
3. Add the carrots, zucchini, and acorn squash and return to a boil. Reduce the heat slightly, cover, and cook for about 20 minutes until the vegetables are tender but not mushy. Remove 2 cups of the cooking liquid and set aside. Season as needed.
4. Add the chickpeas and preserved lemons (if using). Cook for 2 to 3 minutes, and turn off the heat.
5. In a medium pan, bring the remaining 3 cups of water to a boil over high heat. Stir in the couscous, cover, and turn off the heat. Let the couscous rest for 10 minutes. Drizzle with 1 cup of reserved cooking liquid. Using a fork, fluff the couscous.
6. Mound it on a large platter. Drizzle it with the remaining cooking liquid. Remove the vegetables from the pot and arrange on top. Serve the remaining stew in a separate bowl.

Kushari

Ingredients:

<u>For sauce</u>

- 2 tablespoons olive oil
- 2 garlic cloves, minced
- 1 (16-ounce) can tomato sauce
- ¼ cup white vinegar
- ¼ cup Harissa, or store-bought
- 1/8 teaspoon salt

<u>For rice</u>

- 1 cup olive oil
- 2 onions, thinly sliced
- 2 cups dried brown lentils
- 4 quarts plus ½ cup water
- 2 cups short-grain rice
- 1 teaspoon salt
- 1-pound short elbow pasta
- 1 (15-ounce) can chickpeas

Directions:

<u>For sauce</u>

1. In a saucepan over medium heat, heat the olive oil.
2. Add the garlic and cook for 1 minute.

3. Stir in the tomato sauce, vinegar, harissa, and salt. Increase the heat to bring the sauce to a boil. Reduce the heat to low and cook for 20 minutes or until the sauce has thickened. Remove and set aside.

<u>For rice</u>

1. Line a plate with paper towels and set aside.
2. In a large pan over medium heat, heat the olive oil.
3. Add the onions and cook for 7 to 10 minutes, stirring often, until crisp and golden. Transfer the onions to the prepared plate and set aside. Reserve 2 tablespoons of the cooking oil. Reserve the pan.
4. In a large pot over high heat, combine the lentils and 4 cups of water. Bring to a boil and cook for 20 minutes. Drain, transfer to a bowl, and toss with the reserved 2 tablespoons of cooking oil. Set aside. Reserve the pot.
5. Place the pan you used to fry the onions over medium-high heat and add the rice, 4½ cups of water, and the salt to it. Bring to a boil. Reduce the heat to low, cover the pot, and cook for 20 minutes. Turn off the heat and let the rice rest for 10 minutes.6.
6. In the pot used to cook the lentils, bring the remaining 8 cups of water, salted, to a boil over high heat. Drop in the pasta and cook for 6 minutes or according to the package instructions. Drain and set aside.

7. To assemble: Spoon the rice onto a serving platter. Top it with the lentils, chickpeas, and pasta. Drizzle with the hot tomato sauce and sprinkle with the crispy fried onions.

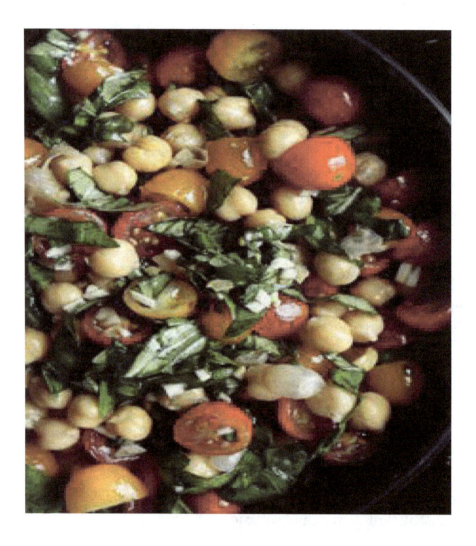

Bulgur with Tomatoes and Chickpeas

Ingredients:

- ½ cup olive oil
- 1 onion, chopped
- 6 tomatoes
- 2 tablespoons tomato paste
- 2 cups water
- 1 tablespoon Harissa
- 1/8 teaspoon salt
- 2 cups coarse bulgur
- 1 (15-ounce) can chickpeas

Directions:

1. In a heavy-bottomed pot over medium heat, heat the olive oil.
2. Add the onion and sauté for 5 minutes.
3. Add the tomatoes with their juice and cook for 5 minutes.
4. Stir in the tomato paste, water, harissa, and salt. Bring to a boil.
5. Stir in the bulgur and chickpeas. Return the mixture to a boil. Reduce the heat to low, cover the pot, and cook for 15 minutes. Let rest for 15 minutes before serving.

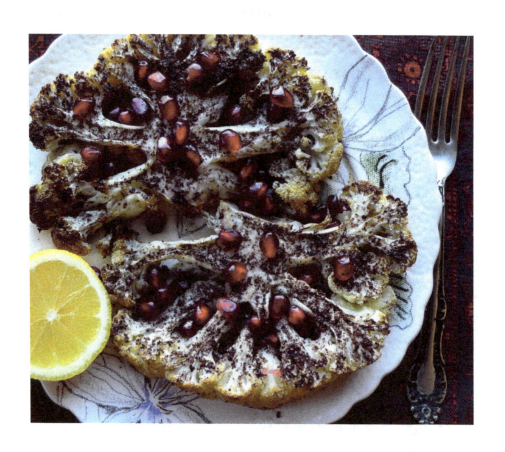

Cauliflower Steaks with Olive Citrus Sauce

Ingredients:

- 2 large heads cauliflowers
- 1/3 cup extra-virgin olive oil
- ¼ teaspoon kosher salt
- 1/8 teaspoon black pepper
- Juice of 1 orange
- Zest of 1 orange
- ¼ cup black olives
- 1 tablespoon Dijon mustard
- 1 tablespoon red wine vinegar
- ½ teaspoon ground coriander

Directions:

1. Preheat the oven to 400°F. Line a baking sheet with parchment paper or foil.
2. Cut off the stem of the cauliflower so it will sit upright. Slice it vertically into four thick slabs. Place the cauliflower on the prepared baking sheet. Drizzle with the olive oil, salt, and black

3. pepper. Bake for about 30 minutes, turning over once, until tender and golden brown.
4. In a medium bowl, combine the orange juice, orange zest, olives, mustard, vinegar, and coriander; mix well.
5. Serve the cauliflower warm or at room temperature with the sauce.

Pistachio Mint Pesto Pasta

Ingredients:

- 8 ounces whole-wheat pasta
- 1 cup fresh mint
- ½ cup fresh basil
- 1/3 cup unsalted pistachios, shelled
- 1 garlic clove, peeled
- ½ teaspoon kosher salt
- Juice of ½ lime
- 1/3 cup extra-virgin olive oil

Directions:

1. Cook the pasta according to the package directions. Drain, reserving ½ cup of the pasta water, and set aside.
2. In a food processor, add the mint, basil, pistachios, garlic, salt, and lime juice. Process until the pistachios are coarsely ground. Add the olive oil in a slow, steady stream and process until incorporated.
3. In a large bowl, mix the pasta with the pistachio pesto; toss well to incorporate. If a thinner, more saucy consistency is desired, add some of the reserved pasta water and toss well.

CPSIA information can be obtained
at www.ICGtesting.com
Printed in the USA
BVHW010223130421
604808BV00014B/158

Pistachio Mint Pesto Pasta

Ingredients:

- 8 ounces whole-wheat pasta
- 1 cup fresh mint
- ½ cup fresh basil
- 1/3 cup unsalted pistachios, shelled
- 1 garlic clove, peeled
- ½ teaspoon kosher salt
- Juice of ½ lime
- 1/3 cup extra-virgin olive oil

Directions:

1. Cook the pasta according to the package directions. Drain, reserving ½ cup of the pasta water, and set aside.
2. In a food processor, add the mint, basil, pistachios, garlic, salt, and lime juice. Process until the pistachios are coarsely ground. Add the olive oil in a slow, steady stream and process until incorporated.
3. In a large bowl, mix the pasta with the pistachio pesto; toss well to incorporate. If a thinner, more saucy consistency is desired, add some of the reserved pasta water and toss well.

CPSIA information can be obtained
at www.ICGtesting.com
Printed in the USA
BVHW010223130421
604808BV00014B/158